COMPLETE DETOXIFICATION WITH VITAMINS

INCREASE YOUR HEALTH WITH WATER-SOLUBLE AND LIPOSOLUBLE VITAMINS, IMPROVE YOUR SKIN, YOUR HAIR, YOUR NAILS AND YOUR APPEARANCE

Jessy M. Brown

Table of Contents

Introduction

Vitamins are essential nutrients, which are part of a necessary process that helps release energy from the foods within their composition and from those consumed to keep the skin, nerves and red blood cells in a constant rejuvenating mode.

The two types of vitamin groups would be classified as fat-soluble vitamins and water-soluble vitamins. The fat-soluble vitamins are vitamins A, D, E and K and all of them are generally found in the fat content of foods. Sources of these can also be found in food products such as vegetable oils, nuts, egg yolks, fish oil, whole grains, and intense green leafy vegetables.

Water-soluble vitamins come in the form of vitamin B, C and B complexes. It contains elements such as thiamine, riboflavin, niacin, folate, biotin and pantothenic acid which are all that the body needs to carry out specific functions to ensure optimal functioning of all body systems.

All these vital ingredients that the body needs and cannot get from the daily diet can be obtained by taking the appropriate combinations and amounts of multivitamins and mineral supplements. However, care should be taken when taking these vitamins and minerals, as some of them do not work well together and for some body systems they may end up being stored and eventually cause toxic conditions. This is especially true because other medications are being taken at the same time.

Vitamin deficiencies

Vitamin intake has not yet reached the ideal where anyone can meet the body's daily needs on a regular basis. Some of the reasons include the high cost of supplements and minerals, inappropriate diet plans, the lack of nutritious food intake, the lack of availability of fresh food products such as fresh vegetables and fruits and, of course, the choice of unhealthy foods that always prevails in consumption.

> ## ➤ *The Risks*

Vitamin deficiencies can contribute to a large number of diseases and also to the lack of optimal body functions. These can be clearly shown in the person's inability to function daily with mental acuity and the precise and precise physical execution of functions, and the presence of frequent episodes of fatigue.

The high-risk groups most likely to suffer from vitamin deficiencies would be the elderly, adolescents, young or pregnant and lactating women, alcoholics, cigarette smokers, vegetarians, people on an empty stomach or in dietary interventions, people who abuse laxatives, users of contraceptives and analgesics and other drugs for chronic diseases, and people with specific disorders of the gastrointestinal tract.

In addition to these people who live hectic lifestyles or have very little physical activity in their daily schedules, they will also be another group that will most likely suffer from vitamin deficiencies.

Some of the most pronounced deficiencies, such as vitamin A deficiency, are known to be the leading cause of preventable blindness, disease and serious infections affecting children. Lack of vitamin D in the diet could lead to fragile bones, as this vitamin is essential for bone formation and growth.

Vitamin E supplementation will play an important role in supporting brain growth and cardiovascular and respiratory functions. Lack of vitamin B is also detrimental to the overall health of the body's system, as it is the main element in the manufacture of red blood cells that keeps the nervous system functioning efficiently.

What types of vitamins are there?

Obtaining all of the body's nutrient requirements can be done through daily or regulated vitamin intake. There are two basic categories of vitamins that are water-soluble and fat-soluble.

The water-soluble vitamins would be vitamins B and C, while the fat-soluble vitamins would be vitamins A, D, E and K. Water-soluble vitamins would be eliminated from the body system on a regular basis, hence the need to consume daily doses of this type of group.

Fat-soluble vitamins are often stored in the body's fatty tissues, hence the need to use them to avoid unnecessary retentions that could cause negative medical complications.

➢ *Types of vitamins*

The following is a list of some of the most prominent vitamins that are commonly recommended and consumed:

Vitamin A - this plays a role in improving eyesight and maintaining healthy skin conditions. It can be obtained from eggs, milk, apricots, spinach and sweet potatoes.

Vitamin B - This particular vitamin has other breakdown sections including B1, B2, B6, B12, niacin, folic acid, biotin, and pantothenic acid.

They generate the energy the body needs for daily functions and also actively participate in the production of red blood cells that carry oxygen throughout the body system.

These can come from wheat, oats, fish, shellfish, leafy vegetables, milk, yogurt, beans, and peas.

Vitamin C - this vitamin helps strengthen gums and muscles, while helping to heal wounds and overcome infections. Its main source is tomatoes, cabbages, broccoli and strawberries.

Vitamin D - strengthens bones and teeth and also aids in the absorption of calcium. It can be found in fish, egg yolk, milk, and some other dairy products.

Vitamin E - takes care of lung functions and also helps in the formation of red blood cells. It can be found in nuts, green leaves, oats, wheat and milk.

Vitamins in food

Although natural foods are rich in a variety of vitamins, it should be noted that many of these vitamins are lost due to storage, cooking and handling.

Therefore, it is important to carefully care for natural foods so that the integrity of the product remains intact. Some vitamins should not be taken with other medications, and some vitamin combinations are also not adequate.

For best results, a medical professional should be consulted so that an appropriate combination can be designed to suit the person's needs and wants.

> ### Sources

The following is a general summary of the various food sources of the most common vitamins:

Vitamin A - beef liver, fatty fish, milk, egg yolks and cheese.

Vitamin C - oranges, Brussels sprouts, strawberries, broccoli, kale.

Vitamin D - canned sardines, mackerel, herring, shrimp, fortifies milk.

Beta-carotene - peaches, sweet potatoes, carrots, spinach, acorn squash.

Vitamin E - wheat germ oil, safflower oil, sunflower oil, spinach, wheat germ, in other words, eggs and oats.

Vitamin K - turnip greens, broccoli, cabbage, spinach and beef liver.

Vitamin B1 (thiamine) - wheat germ, ham, beef liver, peanuts, green peas, pork, and brown rice.

Vitamin B2 (riboflavin) - beef liver, milk, yoghurt, avocados, kale and yeast.

Vitamin B3 (niacin) - chicken, salmon, beef, peanut butter, potatoes, sunflower seeds and prunes.

Vitamin B% (pantothenic acid) - beef liver, eggs, avocados, mushrooms, milk, nuts, and green vegetables.

Vitamin B6 (pyridoxine) - bananas, avocados, beef, chicken, fish, seeds and cabbage.

Vitamin B12 (cobalamin) - beef liver, clams, tuna, yogurt, milk, cheese and eggs.

Folic acid (vitamin BC) - beef liver, spinach, orange juice, romaine lettuce, beets, carrots, egg yolk, avocados and apricots.

Biotin - beef liver, almonds, peanut butter, eggs, oat bran, unpolished rice, meat and dairy products.

How to choose the right vitamins?

Even the most comprehensive diet plan often does not meet all the daily nutritional intake needs of everyone, from children to adults. Some of the reasons for these imbalances are, for example, inadequate diet plans, excessive consumption of fast and convenient foods, and the fact that there are not enough fruits and vegetables to occupy a prominent place in the daily diet.

This is where the nutritional support of vitamins can be helpful. However, it would be crazy to assume it and all vitamins are suitable for everyone equally.

Some considerations must be made, such as lifestyle, availability of natural food products, individual health problems and other factors that play a dominant role in deciding the right vitamin to be consumed.

➢ *The selection*

Almost all medical experts still believe that the best source of vitamins is still natural foods, but due to a variety of reasons it is not always possible to get the daily requirement through this single source, therefore, the need to create a balance with the addition of vitamins in the daily nutrition regimen.

Most experts advocate the consumption of a daily dose of multivitamins, which is usually sufficient to adequately treat any deficiency, if the individual is already on a fairly healthy diet plan.

However, if the individual is already taking another medication to treat other medical conditions, it may not be an appropriate option to consider. Some vitamins do not react well to certain medications and this should be carefully considered to avoid any adverse effects to the body system while taking both without consulting a physician.

Breastfeeding women and pregnant women need a whole range of other vitamins to help balance any deficiencies due to the conditions in which they find themselves. Similarly, those in the older group may also need higher doses of vitamins or a different variety compared to the younger group, since older people tend to eat less and their daily diets usually do not contain all the necessary vitamins the body needs.

Vitamins for babies... Is it safe?

It has long been established that most breastfed babies actually have a complete, healthy and balanced diet and that parents do not have to worry about lack of food.

However, in recent years, research has shown that many pregnant and breastfeeding women do not follow a complete and healthy eating plan for themselves, which in turn affects the overall health of the baby.

In some cases it may be necessary to supplement a children's diet plan with specifically identified vitamins. Under no circumstances should a baby be fed over-the-counter vitamins without the approval of an experienced doctor.

> ➢ **For the Baby**

Some babies may need vitamin D supplements if their daily milk intake is less than 32 ounces of formula or breast milk, although it may be a little more difficult to measure the amount of milk consumed if it is not expressed in a bottle....

Premature babies and babies born with medical problems may need the help of vitamin supplements to help them fight to stay healthy and grow accordingly.

This also applies to the mother who has had previous medical problems, so she may not be able to provide all of the complete and necessary vitamins to the fetus when carrying the child to term.

Some mothers who follow a vegetarian diet during pregnancy may also need to consider some form of vitamin supplement for the baby sometime after the baby's first 6 months of life.

Some popular recommendations that doctors may suggest for babies include a supplement of iron, vitamin D, vitamin B12, and DHA, which is an important omega-3 supplement.

However, none of them should be incorporated into a baby's diet without the specific recommendation of a physician. Even so, it should only be done after a thorough medical examination has been carried out...

Vitamins for adults

Most adults today are not able to get the full nutritional needs of their daily diet plan for a variety of reasons. Even if the healthiest food choices are prepared and consumed daily, this does not necessarily mean that the optimal nutritional intake is achieved.

This may be due to the fact that some methods of cultivation and preservation, and even cooking or preparation methods, contribute to the negative effects on the integrity of the natural foodstuff itself, so that when it is ready for consumption most of the value of its original content has been lost.

Lifestyles also affect the body's nutritional needs, so only after taking all these factors into account can the ideal supplement be chosen.

➤ *For adults*

Ideally, the daily diet should contain all food groups, such as fruit groups, vegetable groups, nut and grain sources, meat and protein sources, and legume groups. However, for one reason or another, it is almost always impossible to create a balanced diet with all these groups included daily.

Deciding to take doses of vitamins as a substitute for adequate food intake is also not something to consider, as this is definitely not adequate for the daily needs of the body.

All adults should have all of the following vitamins included in their daily diet plans:

Vitamin A - for daily cell reproduction and optimal immune conditions to fight disease. This is also necessary for the formation of some hormones, aids in vision and bone growth, maintaining the health of the skin, hair and mucous membranes.

Vitamin B - this is for the production and maintenance of energy levels, the conversion of carbohydrates into energy sources, the optimal functioning of the heart muscle and nervous systems.

Vitamin B2 - important for the body's growth and reproductive capacities, along with the growth of red blood cells and the release of energy from carbohydrates.

Vitamins for the elderly

For the older person, creating and maintaining an ideal diet plan for that age group can be challenging. This is because there are many connective factors that dictate the well-being of those in this age group.

These factors may include the use of medications for certain ailments, lack of energy or interest in preparing nutritious meals, especially if it is for the consumption of a single person, lack of access to the purchase of fresh produce, and financial restrictions.

However, serious consideration should be given to ensuring that the elderly group tries to follow a diet plan that is balanced and nutritious. This can be done with the help of vitamins to supplement any deficiencies found in the person's diet plan or medical makeup.

> ## *For the Elderly*

The following are some of the vitamins that ideally should be considered for consumption by this particular age group:

Vitamin D - this vitamin will help the body absorb calcium as this age group is more prone to osteoporosis. This vitamin also helps in the fight against most heart disease, which is something this age group is susceptible to.

All the various types of vitamin B - the elderly group often has trouble creating their own stomach acid, which is essential to being able to help turn certain foods into elements that the body can use.

In addition to helping in this area, it also helps keep the brain in optimal condition so that memory loss and other brain-delibiting diseases are kept at bay.

Vitamin K - this is especially useful to combat any onset of Alzheimer's disease.

It also helps the blood clot more effectively, as most older people attest that they have significant problems controlling bleeding. In some cases, it has also been observed that this vitamin may help improve opteoporosis conditions.

Watch out for the vitamin overdose!

There are many reasons why people tend to take a vitamin overdose, and in some cases they don't even realize this condition until it appears on some medical exam that it is caused by a disease. The overdose may be due to a number of reasons and most are simply because the person is careless or misinformed.

Taking vitamin supplements without proper medical supervision is also not recommended because some vitamins do not react well to other medications that the individual may be taking for certain medical conditions.

Taking these vitamin supplements may cause other medications to mutate or at least become ineffective in treating the disease for which treatment was prescribed.

This, of course, could result in a very dangerous situation for the individual. There are also some vitamins that are known to eliminate the effects of other vitamins when taken together. Following the prescribed dosage on the package is also very important so that any deviation can result in an overdose, especially when taken extra just to compensate for missed sessions.

Another way to ensure that an individual is not likely to overdose on vitamins is to have periodic blood tests, as any negative elements will clearly appear in the reports made from the remains.

Conclusion

Conclusion of the meeting

Taking vitamin supplements just because it's the right thing to do is not a good enough reason to start with this regiment. Taking vitamins without considering the individual's overall lifestyle is also not a good idea.

For some who take vitamin supplements it is done so, instead of adequate food intake, and this is also not prudent. All of these scenarios can and usually lead to the body not being able to absorb the vitamin fast enough and thus retain it for possible negative medical complications, or to it being wasted, since it is simply eliminated from the body system without using...

I hope you're on your way to a better understanding of vitamins now.

Now yes, I wish you the best in your results, and remember, everything is practical; theory without action is of no use to you. It brings everything you learn into real life.

(you can find it by scanning this code)

A big hug, your friend, Jessy!

By the way, when you achieve your results little by little, I highly recommend you, if you want to learn much more about methods of losing weight, my book, on "HOW TO DO A COMPLETE NATURAL DEINTOXICATION", is a book that I'm sure will help you a lot on your way to "good health". Without further ado, you can find it in the Amazon search engine, like: "How to do a complete natural detox" or looking for my name, like: "Jessy M. Brown"... Once again I wish you success in your results!

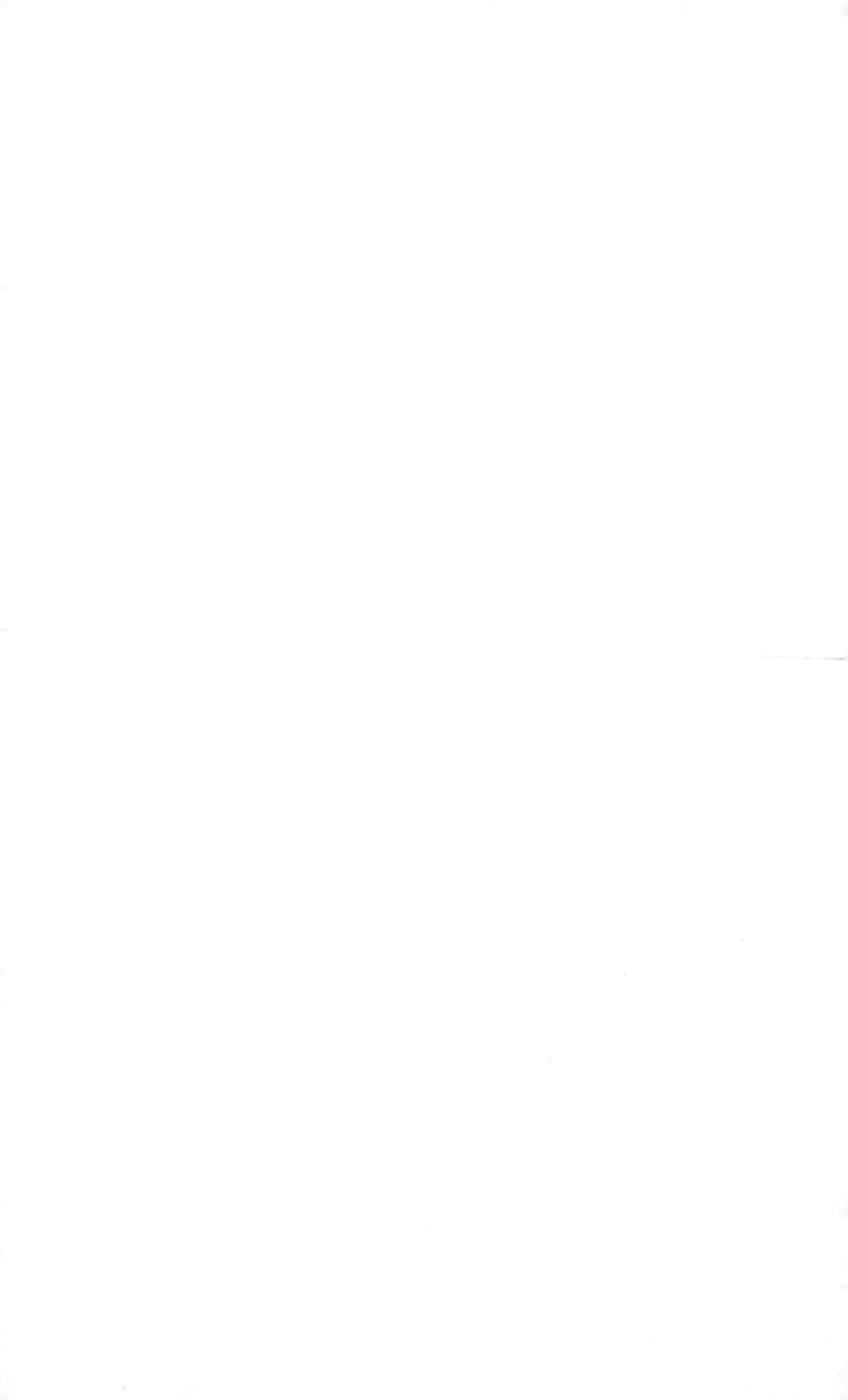